Chapter 1

The Process:

What's the Deal?

Welcome to Chapter 1, My name's Rebekah Van Natta but a lot of people call me RVN. I am a personal trainer and certified integrated reflexologist. I've been involved in health and fitness my whole life, thanks to my wonderful parents. As an adult I started teaching my first indoor cycling class at age 19 and went on from there. I've been working in the fitness industry for over 9 years, and I have been practicing and studying in the field of reflexology for the last 5. So let's get into it...you! You didn't buy this book because you weren't ready to take the next step. You consciously thought about changing your routine, making a change in your life to help improve your health and wellness, and ultimately feel and look better in your day to day life. GOOD, then you'll need to know that living a healthy lifestyle is a process and no magical pill or exercise routine will give you the body you want in a week or 10 days. Here's the deal you made a choice today to start reading this book on YOUR HABIT- The Filthy Five, because you made a choice mentally to change your physical lifestyle. This change your making will fade quickly unless you accept that there's a process to it. It's time to put aside any anger, frustration, or negative feelings you have about you,

5 STEPS TO MOTIVATION

5 Weeks to a healthier you

by
Rebekah Van Natta

your lifestyle, your body, your inactivity. It's time now to focus on the process of finding, sustaining, and keeping a long term healthy lifestyle.

Exercise is like therapy, think of why you are reading this book. Why did you decide to buy it in the first place? What was the motive behind it all? You took time out of your day to look up a self help, motivational health book. Then you had to pull a credit card out of your wallet and fill out a form. Now you have to find the time to read the book and follow "The Plan" and "Guide Lines" to help you find a way to live a healthier lifestyle. If you've read this much then I'd say your ready to build a healthier you.

The beginning of this process is accepting where you are, regardless of past failures. If you can't accept where you are then you will never be able to see a positive outcome and it will always hold you back from reaching your goals. The next few chapters will help you follow the process of achieving motivation, which can and will give you results.

Motivation means:
The act or PROCESS of
giving someone a
reason to do

something, it is the CONDITION of being eager to act or work, it is a FORCE of influence that causes someone to do something

That is a powerful definition of a word...Motivation. Now think about why you may feel unmotivated to eat right, exercise, stay active, make time for yourself, do you sleep not enough hours or too many hours? Why is it hard for you to take care of yourself? What is the motive to an unhealthy lifestyle vs a healthy lifestyle? Are you lazy? Are you scared, do you not know how? Do you not want to put in the effort? Are you thinking about yourself instead of maybe your children or spouse? What is your motive for the actions you've been taking, and what is the motive behind the change you want to take place now? These questions will identify exactly why you are doing what you are doing! What is your motivation for seeking a healthier you? I found my motivation in my mother, which I will go into detail later on. Below I have provided space for you to write down a few things that should help keep you focused on the vision you want to commit to.

Why a Healthier Lifestyle?

Why Now?

What Motivates You?

Make sure you look back to these three questions when you feel you've lost motivation. It's important to stay focused on your motivation while in the beginning of the process, because it is not a routine you are use to. Many people give up too easily because they forget their motivation and let fear distract them from accomplishing their goal. It's time to get rid of fear and go full out. Accept that this journey is a long one, it may be bumpy and rough at first. I promise it will get easier along the way. If you stay true to the motive behind the reason you will find it much easier to get through. It seems like steps right now because...well it is, but soon enough the steps become a daily fabric of your life and there is no thinking or fearing of what or what not to do. That is the realistic and attainable goal ahead for you! Along with the next few chapters of this book, there are 15 exercises and 5 recipe guidelines that will easily guide you to fall into a healthier routine. Following the exercises and implementing a few new healthy recipes can help break up the habit of the unhealthy lifestyle you've fallen into. Discipline takes action. If you want change then you will have to use your actions, to make that change a long lasting one. Consistency is the key role in the discipline, finding the consistency with doing your workouts and eating better is vital especially in the beginning. As you know consistency and balance are the key to life. If you have felt out of balance with your diet and your health, then you have fallen out of the consistency of life. Maybe your consistently inconsistent with life. It happens, it's okay, but there's a point you've hit revealing, that now is the time to find that balance in your life again. If you're still reading, then your ready to find the balance and consistency in your life. This will help you to be a healthier and happy you. This is possible because you have already envisioned a healthier you, and are now taking the steps into committing to that vision. I would say now...it's go time!

Chapter 2

Rebekah's Ladder:

Realistic Goals

Welcome to Chapter 2, my ladder on setting Realistic Goals. Let's be honest if you want to lose 20lbs in a week it ain't happening! If you want to set a goal of working out everyday and eating clean for the next few weeks, it probably ain't happening! If you think a juice cleanse or a fad diet is going to help you find the solution to your weight management problem...probably not a good idea! I know we want results fast and we want them the easiest way possible...but it's not realistic. Our society thrives off of what is the fastest way to get things done. Pills, diets, cleanses, detoxes, liposuction, even as extreme as surgeries to shrink your stomach. It goes on and on, we want results and we want them now! Yes, yes, this I know! But really?

According to Peter F. Rovito, MD, FACS - Bariatric Surgeon. Statistics show that almost 70% or in other words, at 100 pounds overweight the average patient loses almost 70 pounds. And many patients have seen results of well over 80%. "Most patients keep at least 50% of their excess weight off after 10 years." But once you reach your low point called your "nadir", the question is will you start heading in the opposite direction? Unfortunately, it's very likely.

It's difficult for people who do these extreme diets and fads to find long lasting results. It takes skills, the motivation, and discipline to exercise daily and eat right. Needless to say it's best to walk through the process to have long lasting effects rather than lose all your weight and then most likely gain it all back or more.

Put exercise and health on the same spectrum as a relationship. There are many different forms and kinds of relationships, but none the less a relationship is on going and takes effort. In life we have everything from family, to friends, work, career, hobbies and interests. In all those areas of our lives, a relationship has to form in some way or another. You don't just marry the first person you go on a date with...sometimes but rarely. You have to get to know them, and form a relationship with them before marriage and a family can happen. And as we all know, relationships are hard and you have to work at them. You don't get a promotion from going to a job interview...you have to first apply, go through the interview process, get hired, then work and form relationships with the company before anything else can take place. Friendships don't happen over night either! I've been really blessed to have so many childhood friends still current in my life, but through all the years of knowing each one of them we have all had our fights, disagreements, and immaturity we've had to work through. Even now in my adult life, real friendships are hard to find. When you do find a person or group of people that become part of your life, it's because a lot of time has been invested. Hobbies and interests are things that we are either good at or enjoy doing. Just because you like doing something doesn't mean your great at it. There are always new things we are learning with our interests and skills, that we will forever be crafting to make better. So as before a lot of time has to be invested so we can grow and get better at what we like doing. Just remember if all those things in our day to day life are tied into a form of a relationship, then exercise and health need to be too.

You are the author of your body

Rebekah Van Natta

Don't lose sight of the fact, that you only get one body for the rest of your life. I use to say to my clients "You are the author of your body". You need to have a relationship with your body. If you feel disconnected from your body, then it's time to start forming and working on that relationship now! So how do we find simplicity in the craziness of our every day lives? Even more so, simplicity in finding the time for ourselves? Well it starts with a choice, then a commitment, then it requires you to follow through. This commitment can become routine. There is a need to have a healthy view of what you can become in your mind. If you do not have this, it will be difficult to achieve. In the routine you will find the time to commit to building the healthier you. Just like I said in Chapter 1, you cannot start building anything until you fully accept where you are. The routine will feel hard, and difficult at times. You may want to stop at times, or even tell yourself, "I'll start this next week". But then your going to look at the three questions you answered in Chapter 1 and remember why you made the commitment to change.

Here are a few ideas and questions you should ask yourself

- What are my interests?
- What activities do I enjoy?

Swimming, Running, Walking, Jogging, Biking, Lifting, Spinning, Yoga, Stretching, Dancing, Hiking, Group Exercise, working out alone, Partner Workouts, Stairs, Roller-skating, Body weighted workouts, Cardio Driven Workouts, Martial Arts, Kickboxing, Zumba, Boxing, Thai-Chi, Rock Climbing

- How many days do I want to commit to working out?
- How many hours a day do I want to commit to working out?
- What foods can I void or add in?
- Do I drink enough water?

Keep in mind that the questions above need to be answered realistically, you can always increase the number of days and hours when you are ready to. Just start somewhere! I'll help you:

Beginner: 2xWeek for 30Min a day
Moderate: 3/4xWeek for 30Min-1 Hour a day

Start with something that will get you excited enough to follow through with this commitment. Your excitement will grow, and your workouts and your healthy eating will grow. Soon enough you will feel the difference in your body, your mood, your mind that it will excite you to get up and do your workout and eat fairly clean. This is not about perfection, because let's face it we are all FAR from perfect! It's about balance and the willingness to submit your bad habits over to good habits. Good habits that will give you long lasting effects for the rest of your life. Habits that you can be proud about, excited about, and happy about. It's all very self rewarding once you get to the point you're not achy, or bloated, over weight, heavy, tired, exhausted, unmotivated! Climb the ladder don't try to jump to the top. No matter how quickly you want to get there you will fall down if you jump. So stay steady climbing the ladder, take your time, be realistic and stay committed to the choices that your wanting to make. Pushing for bigger results and bigger goals in a short amount of time can be discouraging and also set you back. So when I say "The Ladder" I'm also saying "Steps". Take one step at a time, don't get discouraged, set small and attainable goals and from there go bigger. Trust me I want you to get crazy and say I'm going to run a marathon or that your going to cut out all sugars. Realistically that is not a healthy choice at the beginning. Stay true to what you know you can handle, then later down the road get crazy!

> *"When it is obvious that the goals cannot be reached,*
>
> *don't adjust the goals, adjust the action steps."*
>
> *Confucius*

A little bit about my personal ladder and change. In 2010 my mother Sue, passed away from breast cancer. In honor of my mother I wanted to do something for her. Something that she loved doing, something that could keep her legacy alive. She was a marathoner so I thought a half marathon would be a good start. I absolutely hated running, I was a sprinter and triple-jumper in high school and 200 meters was as far as I enjoyed running. But I was motivated to do something in honor of my mother. Mom ran for The Leukemia Society for over 13 years. She raised hundreds of thousands of dollars running to help find a cure for Leukemia. She had a passion and a joy for helping and serving others. It was through running, raising money, and bringing awareness that she served and helped others. I told myself that I'd run 3 days a week and each day I'd run 3 miles. That's doe-able, attainable and I didn't care how long it took me, I was just going to commit to 3 miles. Whether it was walking it, running it, or dreading it! Running 3 miles now is a piece of cake, but when I started it felt like the longest run of my life! I wanted to stop, give up, say well, "I'll just run a 5k in honor of her" which is 3 miles and call it a day! But my motivation was my mother, and she kept me strong in my runs. I felt her with me as I do now every step I take. I can hear her voice encouraging me, cheering me, and motivating me to keep pushing and keep going. It's been almost 6 years and she is still my drive, my force, my motivation. I not only did several half marathons, but went even crazier and started doing Tri-athlons. There were even more challenges with tri's that went above and beyond the running. Learning first how to swim, staying disciplined with it. Learning how to ride a road bike, learning the gears and then finding my stride. Overcoming the fears of the ocean waves and the ocean swims. It was a huge learning curve for me, and a challenge that I had fully accepted no matter what the outcome. I was motivated! It was through the process "The Ladder", that I was able to accomplish what I wanted to accomplish. I set attainable goals that weren't too overwhelming but challenging enough. It was something I had to be patient with, and work very hard at. Yes, I got frustrated, yes I wanted to stop...but I didn't. I was also very fortunate to have my twin sister push and teach me along the way. She was already into several half marathons and had also completed a few tri-athlons. I had a mentor, a coach, a friend. Read on to the next chapter to find out more about having that accountability that I had.

Chapter 3
Accountability: Make an Announcement

'

As you read in Chapter 2 commitments are hard, relationships are hard, and change is hard! The best way to stay true to the things that you want or need in life is someone or a group of individuals there to make sure you stay on track! You need accountability, you need someone to hold you accountable for the actions your wanting to take. It sounds kind of silly, but it's the truth. Any time I wanted change, I reached out to a group of individuals to hold me accountable for the actions I was wanting to take. Anytime I felt I was about to fall or steer away from my goals, I would have that support system to fall back on. A very important man in my life (My father, Will) told me many times growing up, "If your going to be a man, be a man of your word". Although I'm not a man, what he was trying to instil in me was to have integrity be a person of honor. I try to incorporate what my father told me into my life daily, and that includes with following through with what I say I'm going to do. It's not as easy as it sounds, but with a support group it can help keep you true to my fathers saying.

Finding people to hold you accountable can sometimes be challenging. But, you can also make a public announcement telling friends, co-workers, and family that you are setting a goal with a date. You can keep them posted on your journey every step of the way. This way when you don't post or say anything at least one person is going to ask you, "So how are your workouts coming a long? Have you tried any new recipes?". You'll feel uplifted by the support, encouraged, and motivated to keep going. There's a ripple effect when people see you doing something challenging to better yourself. Most likely they will want to get on board and do it too. You'll find motivation in the pure fact that you are motivating others. It's a win, win really! Here are 6 ways to stay on track:

6 Ways to Stay On Track

1. Tell Someone
- Family
- Co-Workers
- Friends
- Therapist
- Online Support Group
- Schedule Check-In's
- Phone
- Email
- Text
- Facebook or other forms of Social Media

2. Go Public
- Post Your goals on Facebook
- Share weekly or monthly updates on Twitter
- Start a blog about your journey
- Keep a video or diary on You-Tube

3. Get a Workout Buddy
- Set a specific day/time to workout with a partner 1 or 2 times a week, so you know that you both are relying on each other to follow through with the workout and fully commit to it.

4. Sign a Contract
- You may think this is silly, BUT write out an actual contract stating your goals. How you will achieve them, your rewards or consequences for following or not following your routine, and have a family member or friend sign your contract as a witness.

5. Put that Money Down
- No one likes losing money, commit to paying a friend, family member, or co-worker X amount of dollars if you don't achieve a particular goal. Or give a friend a certain amount of money and

earn it back for every goal you accomplish. If you don't achieve your goals, well then your friend get's to keep your money.

6. Sign up for a Race/Event
   I personally love this one, this is what I do. Sign up for a 5k, 10k, ½ or full marathon, a Mud Run, a Tri-athlon, or any kind of race/event. Registering for race can be quite motivational within itself. You can sign up with a team, raise money, and help organizations in finding a solution to so many problems and illnesses we have in this world. You have a team to train with so you will always have a group of supporters and on top of that your making a difference in the world for simply running or racing.

- Team in Training- Benefiting the Leukemia &Lymphoma Society
- Susan G Koman & Pink Streak Team- Benefiting Breast Cancer Research & Support
- American Cancer Society- Benefiting Cancer Research
- Autism Peaks- Benefiting Autism Research

- Legs for Lou Gehrig's Disease-Benefiting ALS Research
- Run to Remember- Benefiting the Alzheimer's Association
- Bike MS- Benefiting Multiple Sclerosis

These are a few organizations, but the list is endless. Look up online different groups in your area or run in honor of someone you know or knew that is going through some type of illness.

So try something that will help you be accounted for! We are all different in the way we think, feel, and react. Find the right way to help you stay on track. You might fail a few times, but keep trying to find a way that really works for you! The results will happen but first you have to commit to the change and focus on the change.

"If you focus on results, you will never change.

If you focus on change, you will get results"

Jack Dixon

So there it is, focus on the change and the results will follow!

Chapter 4
Positivity:
Put a Smile on it

So here we are, we've identified the problem, were setting realistic goals, and we're finding ways to stay on track. Now it's time to put a smile on it. You have to stay positive on this journey. Life is hard enough, why make it more difficult? Complaining will get you no where and fighting yourself will only keep you in a frustrated stressful state. You've made it this far, now you need to stay positive and keep your head up. A lot of what we have already discussed should help keep you in a more positive state. But remember you are the only one that has the key to unlock your own happiness. There will be times when you feel you will want to beat yourself up. Therefore, allowing yourself to tap into a negative mindset. It maybe for not following through with your goals. It could be from falling back into unhealthy eating habits, or not taking the time out to exercise as you had planned. But here's the thing, you always have a choice. Everyday is a new day, start with a positive attitude it will get you further throughout your day. It will take practice just like everything else in life. The positivity will take you further if you just give into it. It's hard to believe it, but positive and negative thinking are very contagious. By contagious I mean, it can be on a subconscious level, through words, thoughts, your feelings, and even your body language. Think about a time when you were in a crappy negative mood. Did you recognize how maybe nothing ever went your way, and if felt like no one was ever around? When you are positive it's obvious people would rather want to be around that, and secondly you are more likely to get the help you need without even asking. What does this have to do with fitness? I'm getting there! Here's the thing, negative thoughts, words, and attitude, all create unhappy feelings, moods, and behaviors. I bet you didn't know that there is scientific proof that when your mind is negative, poisons are released into your blood which automatically causes more unhappiness and negativity. This is a for sure way towards failure, to frustrations, and disappointments. I'm sorry but I don't have time for that, do you? Just like the ladder to realistic goals, positivity has its own ladder. The change will not happen over night, but most importantly you just need to be aware of when a negative thought comes into your mind. Do not let it control you, you have the capability to control your own emotions. This will happen with time, patients, and practice! There are a few ways to help you stay positive.

Tips for Developing a more Positive Attitude

- Choose to be happy. Like I said it's simply a choice, it's not easy but when you start thinking negative thoughts reject them and tap into a happy thought. With practice over time this will get easier
- Look at the good things in your life, again it's a choice and trust me this will take some practice
- Choose to be optimistic. Plus, who likes being around someone who is a pessimist
- Smile More, life is hard enough why go throughout the day with a frown
- Have faith and believe in yourself. If you don't then why should anybody else have faith or believe in you
- Place yourself around others who are happy. You should try to remain around like minded people, it helps keep you on the right course
- See the good in life, and in people. When all you see is the negative it's hard to see the

light, trapping your thoughts into a negative mindset
- Use positive words in your thoughts and words
- Ignore what the world thinks of you and/or what you should or shouldn't be doing/ look like/ act like/ speak like/ have/ don't have
- As a Christian I believe the world is full of lies and false perception. Do not allow the world to define who you are, you are in control of your emotions, you are able to be whoever you choose to be, you choose to live the life you lead
- Let go of anything negative in your life and replace it with something positive in your life past/present/future
- Help and serve others that are less fortunate than you

"A strong, positive self-image is the best possible preparation for success"

Joyce Brothers

Keep in mind all these things are a work in progress, but then again we as humans are always a work in progress. Just like you want your lifestyle to change to be a healthier happier one, staying positive will take time to fall into. Do not get discouraged, and be aware of these emotions that trigger a negative thought. So that when it happens your able to recognize it, and conquer it. Keep this in mind while you set your new goals in living a healthy lifestyle. At home in the gym, at work wherever!

Chapter 5:

Reward Yourself

I think rewards are important! I don't want you to think this means eating ice cream after every workout, but hey it's okay to reward yourself after setting and accomplishing your goals. I love rewards, I love working hard to getting something I want. For example, I train for triathlons, and when I'm training for a certain race I am very headstrong on how much swimming, biking, and running I should be doing. I'm very consistent and I make sure when I train I'm constantly working on strength and endurance. I push myself some days harder than others. On days when I know I will be kicking my butt, I decide it will be a burger and beer or pizza and beer kind of dinner. I will tell you I rarely drink beer or eat pizza, but I'll do it once in a while! After an intense training or race I deserve a darn good meal. Sometimes when I'm setting goals to lean down for a photo shoot or lean down to be lighter while racing, after the race or after the photo-shoot is over, I'll go for some really good ice cream. I love ice cream, but I do not eat it every week or every month! These are just food rewards, there are many others to try both big and small. Here are a few ways to reward yourself after meeting and accomplishing your goals.

Reward Yourself

- Treat yourself to your favorite dessert or entrée
- Make a dinner reservation at a fancy restaurant and get all dressed up
- Get out of town go on a trip or vacation
- Make a special night with your friends or your special somebody
- Go through your closet and donate to the charity of your choice
- Invest in awesome workout clothes, or some new workout shoes
- Sleep in or take a nap
- Schedule a professional photo shoot
- Go pamper yourself
- Massage, Facial, Nails, Hair, Mimosa on the beach, whatever makes you feel good!
- Go out on the town
  - Movies, Concert, Dancing, Sports Game

- Do something you've never done before

Sky diving, Water Rafting, Tubing, Skiing, Bungee Jumping, Surfing, Cooking Class, Pottery Class, Scuba Diving, Snorkeling,

Rock Climbing, Travel to a place you've never been, etc...)

*"Action is the foundational key
to all success"*

Pablo Picasso

The list can be endless; you can find many ways to motivate yourself to be able to pick something on your rewards list to aim for. And the rule goes, if you DO NOT accomplish your goal you DO NOT get your reward. I would encourage you to write down a list of rewards, and make sure they get marked off the list, only when and after your goal is reached. If it's a small goal, make it small reward. If it's a big goal, make it a big reward. This way there's no justifying or lacking on your end, you have worked hard to earn it! The reason your doing this is because you want to feel better right? You want to look good, feel good, and be a happier healthier individual for you and for those you love. Get your family, friends, co-workers, neighbors whoever on bored to help you reach these goals.

Here is what we have covered in this book. It is vital and important that you first figure out what the deal is and accept there's a process to this journey. Start building your ladder and stay realistic with each goal you set. It's vital that you make an announcement about the changes you want in your life, and have someone or a lot of somebodies hold you accountable to the actions and goals your setting. Staying positive is key in allowing change to happen, without it you will fail. Rewarding your self is important because you need to know your work is paying off! I hope this book guides you in finding peace in your journey. Be consistent and remember it is a journey so allow grace along the way. Good luck, find your ladder and take one step at a time!

5 Week Workout Program

Here are your workouts for the next 5 weeks. Follow and make sure you get these in no matter what! Check out videos on my YouTube Channel RVNFIT.

Week 1

10 Minute Workouts
Set your timer for 10 Minutes
You will be doing 3 exercises for time. Keep repeating the 3 exercises, until the 10 minutes is up. These are called AMRAPs = As Many Rounds As Possible

Workout #1

1. 10 Squat + Calf Raise
2. 10 Push Ups
3. 20 Jumping Jacks

Workout #2

1. 20 High Knees
2. 5 Walk out Push ups
3. 10 Bridges + 10 Squeezes/Pulses at top

Workout #3

1. 10 Wide Squat Touch Downs
2. 12 Backward Lunges Alternate
3. 20 Second Plank

Week 2
20 Minute Workouts

Workout #1
Brisk Walk or
Walk/Run
- 4 Min Walk/ 1 Min Jog
- 3 Min Walk/ 2 Min Jog

Workout #2
Walk 5 Minutes, 10 Push Ups + 20
Squats Repeat

Workout #3
Brisk Walk or
Walk/Run
- 4 Min Walk/ 1 Min Jog
- 3 Min Walk/ 2 Min Jog

Week 3

10 Minute Workouts

Workout #1

1.) 30 Low Jumping Jacks
2.) 10 Walk Outs + Push Up
3.) 20 Side Reaches

Workout #2

1.) 20 Side Jump Lunges
2.) 30 Second Plank
3.) 10 Bicep Curl to Shoulder Press

Workout #3

1.) 5 Burpees
   - Modify by walking back lowering down to knees and walking feet back to standing
2.) 10 Reverse Fly
3.) 20 Twist Jumps

Week 4
20 Minute Workouts

Workout #1
Walk/Run
- 3 Min Walk/ 2 Min Jog

Workout #2
Walk 5 min, 20 Walking Forward Lunges
+ 5 Burpees, Repeat

Workout #3
Walk/Run
- 3 Min Walk/ 2 Min Jog

Week 5
30 Minute Workouts

Workout #1
10 Minute Walk/Jog Warm Up
10 Minute AMRAP
1.)20 Squat Jumps/ Or Regular Squats
2.)10 Walk Out + Push Up
3.) 30 Sec-1 Min Plank
10 Minute Walk/Jog Cool Down

Workout #2
10 Minute Walk/Jog Warm Up
10 Minute AMRAP
1.) 20 Side Jump Lunge OR Walk Through
2.) 10 Super Man's
3.) 20 Bridges
10 Minute Walk/Jog Cool Down

Workout #3
10 Minute Walk/Jog Warm Up
10 Minute AMRAP
1.) 10 Burpees
2.) 10 Bicep Curl to Shoulder Press
3.) 15 Rows
10 Minute Walk/Jog Cool Down

5 You Pick Recipes

These recipes are here to help you incorporate some healthier options and variations of food choices. I'm not asking you to take out anything, just add in one new recipe every week for the next five weeks.

Daily Note

Start adding 1 cup of warm lemon water in the AM every morning on an empty stomach.
Try to limit your portions according to:
Fruits: 1- 1.5 Cup
Veggies: 2-3 Cups
Protein: Palm of Hand 3oz of Meat, Fish, Poultry
Carbs: 1-3 Cups

Warm Lemon Water

And its benefits...
Balances PH Level
Boots your Immune System
Aids in Digestion
Acts as a Natural Diuretic
Hydrates your Lymph System
Aids in Weight Loss
Helps to Purify and Stimulate the Liver

Week 1
Breakfast

Chocolate Mint Shake
1 Scoop Vega Vanilla & Greens Protein
1 Frozen Banana
1Tbsp Unsweetened Cocoa Powder
1-2Cups Almond or Cashew Milk
1 -2Drop DoTerra Peppermint Oil
2-6 Ice Cubes (Depending on how thick
you like your shake/ice cream)
Dash-1/2 Tbsp Truvia to taste (opt for
more sweetness)

If you want to void the banana because
of the starch you can use 1/4 an
avocado instead.

For the Vega Protein & Greens-Vegan
Plant Based Protein
You can order right from my site
rebekahvannatta.com

For the DoTerra Peppermint Oil go to:
www.doterra.com

I promise you will love it! And if you are
not a peppermint fan, just follow the
recipe and take out the peppermint oil!
It's also very easy to make it taste
whatever flavor you like (Strawberry,
blueberry, banana, coffee, cinnamon,

orange, coconut, raspberry, pineapple, etc...)

Option 2

Almond Oatmeal Bowl
1/2Cup Rolled Oats
1Cup Water
Handful of Raspberries
1Tbsp Almond Butter
Splash of Almond or Cashew Milk
1Tbsp Chia Seeds

Option 3

Sweet Energy Boost Yogurt Bowl
1Cup Plain Yogurt
1/2Tbsp Grounded Flaxseed
1/2Tbsp Chia Seeds
1/2Cup Blueberries
1/2 Handful Goji Berries
Drizzle Coconut Oil

Week 2
Build Your Own Salad

Mix and match do whatever you'd like. You can have a different meal everyday, start by picking:

Green Options:
Spinach, Mixed Greens, Arugula, Kale, Cabbage (Red, Green, Napa), Lettuce (Butter, Romaine, Red Leaf, Green Leaf)

Pick 2-3 Veggies:
Carrots, Bell Peppers (Red, Yellow, Orange), Cucumber, Celery, Beets, Zucchini

1 Herb:
Parsley, Cilantro, Basil, Alfalfa

½ Cup Fruit or Less:
Spring: apricots, strawberries, mango, oranges, pineapple
Summer: asian pear, berries, melon, cherries, figs, grapes, nectarines, peaches, plums
Fall: pears, apples, cranberries, grapes, pomegranates
Winter: clementines, grapefruits, oranges, tangerines, kiwi, papaya
Year-round: dried fruits, avocado

1 Protein:
Steak, Chicken, Turkey, Ham, Bacon, Fish/Seafood/Tuna, Garbanzo Beans, Tofu, Black & White, Beans, Hard Boiled Eggs, Any left overs!

Accents:
Pecans, Walnuts, Almonds, Pumpkin/Sunflower Seeds, Edible Flowers

Dressing (Single Serving)
1/4 Lemon Squeezed
1 Clove Garlic Minced
Drizzle Avocado Oil or Olive Oil
Drizzle Balsamic Vinegar (opt)
Dash Salt, Pepper, Dried Basil

Week 3
Build Your Own Dinner

Mix and match do whatever you'd like. You can have a different meal everyday, start by picking:

1 Protein:
Steak, Chicken, Turkey, Ham, Bacon, Fish/Seafood/Tuna, Garbanzo Beans, Tofu, Black & White, Beans, Hard Boiled Eggs

Pick 1-2 Veggies:
Broccoli, Cauliflower, Zucchini, Asparagus, Green Beans, Carrots, Kale, Artichokes
- Squeeze Lemon, 1Tbsp Olive/Avocado Oil & Minced Garlic after steam

1 Herb:
Parsley, Cilantro, Basil, Alfalfa

1 Carbohydrate:
Quinoa, Brown Rice, Sweet Potato, Butternut Squash, Spaghetti squash (1Cup is fine)

Week 4
Simple Snacking

Rice Cakes with Peanut or Almond
Butter

Cottage Cheese & Pineapple

Edamame

Plain Organic Popcorn

Apple

Hard Boil Eggs

Hummus & Veggies

- Take Carrots, Celery, Cucumber, Snow Peas. Throw in plastic cup for quick to go snack and dip

Nut Butter Boat

- Celery or Apple with nut butter & almonds & raisins

Beet Chips with Curried Yogurt

- Mix together 2 tablespoons plain low-fat Greek yogurt and ⅛ to ¼ teaspoon curry powder. Serve with 1 cup beet chips.

Ham and Jicama Wraps

- Dividing evenly, wrap 6 jicama or celery sticks with 3 slices ham. Serve with 1 teaspoon whole-grain mustard for dipping.

Banana, Kale, and Almond Milk
Smoothie

- In a blender, puree 1 medium banana, 1 cup chopped kale, and 1 cup almond milk until smooth.

Whole-Grain Bread with Almond Butter and Peaches

- Spread 2 teaspoons almond butter on 1 slice toasted whole-grain bread. Top with ½ sliced peach.

Week 5
Simple Healthy Desserts

Single Serve Chocolate Cake
Ingredients:
1Tbsp plus 2 tsp cocoa powder
3Tbsp Gluten Free Flour
1/8 tsp salt
2tsp Xylitol or Truvia
1/4 tsp baking powder
pinch uncut stevia OR 1 more Tbsp Xylitol or Truvia
2-3 tsp coconut oil OR applesauce
3Tbsp milk of choice (I used almond milk)
1/2 tsp pure vanilla extract

Recipe:
Combine dry ingredients and mix very, well. Add liquid, stir, then transfer to a little dish, ramekin, or even a coffee mug. Either microwave 30-40 seconds OR cook in a 350F oven for about 14 minutes. If you don't want to eat it straight out of the dish, be sure to spray your dish first then wait for it to cool before trying to remove it.

Chocolate Frosting
Ingredients:
4Tbsp nut butter (I used peanut)
1/2 a large, very ripe banana

2Tbsp
cocoa powder
pinch of salt
pinch of Xylitol, Stevia, or Truvia

Recipe:
Blend everything (including chips, if
using) in a small food processor or
Magic Bullet. If you have a bigger
processor, it might be best to double
the recipe so everything blends more
smoothly. Best to store uneaten frosting
covered in the fridge. Substitution
notes: If you don't like—or can't have—
peanut butter, feel free to try this recipe
with almond butter, cashew butter,
sunbutter, or coconut butter!

Raw Chocolate Fudge Balls
Ingredients:
1 1/2Cups pitted dates
1Tbsp plus 2 tsp cacao or cocoa powder
1/8 tsp salt
optional small handful
chocolate chips
optional cocoa, shredded coconut,
melted chocolate, etc

Recipe:
Combine the first three ingredients (and
chips, if using) in a strong food
processor or Vitamix, and blend until
completely smooth. Scoop into a bowl,

and freeze until the sticky dough is firm enough to roll balls (a half hour or so). Once balls are rolled—either with your hands or a mini cookie scoop—you can roll in the optional cocoa or coconut, or just eat them plain. I stored leftover raw chocolate fudge balls in the freezer to keep them as firm as possible.

Black Bean Brownies

Ingredients:
1 1/2Cups black beans (1 15-oz can, drained and rinsed very well)
2Tbsp cocoa powder
1/2Cup quick oats
1/4 tsp salt
1/3Cup pure maple syrup or agave (or honey, but not for strict vegans.)
pinch uncut stevia OR 2 Tbsp Xylitol/Truvia (or omit and increase maple syrup to 1/2 cup)
1/4Cup coconut
2tsp pure vanilla extract
1/2 tsp baking powder
1/2Cup to 2/3Cup chocolate chips
optional: more chips, for presentation

Recipe:
Preheat oven to 350 F. Combine all ingredients except chips in a good food processor, and blend until completely smooth. Really blend well. A blender works but a food processor could be

better. Stir in the chips, then pour into a greased 8×8 pan. Optional: sprinkle extra chocolate chips over the top. Cook the black bean brownies 15-18 minutes, then let cool at least 10 minutes before trying to cut. If they still look a bit undercooked, you can place them in the fridge overnight and they will magically firm up! Makes 9-12 brownies.

Healthy Ice Cream

Ingredients:
6-8 Bananas
Whatever flavor you want- Chocolate, Peanut Butter, Coffee, Blueberries, Mangos, Strawberries, Cinnamon, Vanilla etc..

Recipe:
To freeze bananas: Peel and slice bananas into 1/2" rounds. Place in a single layer on a parchment-lined baking sheet and freeze for at least 2 hours. (If you plan to keep them in the freezer longer than 2 hours, store the already-frozen rounds in an airtight plastic freezer bag.) Pour frozen banana slices into a food processor. Pulse until the bananas are broken up. You'll need to regularly remove the lid of the food processor and scrape down the sides with a rubber spatula. Then continue to process the bananas.

Once the bananas are creamy, toss in your mix-ins and continue to blend until your mixture is completely creamy. Serve immediately. Do not attempt to re-freeze, because it won't have that same creamy consistency.

Guilt Free Frozen Yogurt

Ingredients:
Plain Non Fat Yogurt
Sliced Almonds
Fresh Sliced Strawberries
Honey or Truvia/Stevia/Xylitol
Cinnamon
Dark Chocolate Chips (opt)
Waffle Cone

Recipe:
Mix up, scoop into waffle cone either enjoy as is or place in the freezer for 30min-1hour! Or enjoy in a bowl!

Note: Remember

Stay consistent and remember, it's not about racing to the finish line. It's about the journey and finding a balance that's sustainable! So enjoy every step of the way into living a healthy lifestyle.

For more info, check **www.rebekahvannatta.com** for new workouts and subscribe to my FREE newsletter where I share with you my health podcasts, workouts, recipes, and life! If you don't follow me on any social media my links are below. Join or subscribe to my pages and my You-Tube channel to stay connected and motivated!

Stay Connected Links:

Instagram @ RVNFIT

Facebook fan page: RVNFIT

Health & Wellness Podcast:
SoundCloud.com- Rebekah Van Natta
iTunes- RVNFIT

Blogger:
www.rvnfit.blogspot.com

Join my FREE newsletter through my website rebekahvannatta.com for fun podcasts, healthy recipes, workouts, and inspirational/motivational tips!

Thank you for watching. Please Subscribe to, like & share my videos on YouTube- RVNFIT

DoTerra Oils-Essential Oils: www.doterra.com